A MOTHER'S GUIDE
FOR MANIFESTING JOY

A MOTHER'S GUIDE FOR MANIFESTING

JOY

Navigating your way through
the postpartum roller coaster

LINDSAY R. JOHNSON

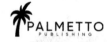

Charleston, SC
www.PalmettoPublishing.com

A Mother's Guide for Manifesting JOY
Copyright © 2021 by Lindsay R. Johnson

First Edition

ISBN: 978-1-64990-976-3

Motherhood is something that comes naturally and joyfully for a lot of women, but not everyone. By going through my own four-year roller coaster of a journey as a new (40-year-old) mom, driven, scared, conditioned, competitive, wanting to be the best I could be; I've learned a lot in the process, to say the least. I've learned how to manifest joy, how to create balance, how to serve myself before others sometimes, and that it is normal to not be that natural super mom that so many others are born to be (and kudos to them!!). My goal with this book is to help. The struggle is real, ladies, and it is okay. You are not alone. There is JOY through this tunnel, and my hope is to steer you back in that direction with energy-based tools, abundant resources, personal and client experiences, laughter, and a whole lot of honest love.

CONTENTS

AUTHOR'S NOTES/ACKNOWLEDGMENT

As I navigate through this book, citing my own experiences and the experiences of others, my goal is to reference as many of the supporters and guides I have encountered as possible. Please do forgive if I have overlooked anyone in the process. This process of diving into this journey and accepting what comes to you takes a sense of freedom and openness, and it cannot necessarily be referenced in totality. With that being said, I do want to thank my own anxiety, postpartum depression, conditioning, and past traumas. Yes, you read that right. Together they have helped mold me into this newly found spiritual Alchemist that I was drawn to be and share. This obviously wouldn't be a journey without them, and I couldn't help others without this experience. For that I am forever grateful. I would also like to thank my dear son Kingston, the reason I am a mother, the King to my wellness. Without him I never would have been able to find my Joy again. I would have never taken this path with my career, grown this much as a person, and written this book. Finally, my husband, my energizer bunny, and full-throttle supporter, who enables me to believe anything is possible. Thank you for always supporting my crazy business ideas and ever-flowing dreams.

I would like to dedicate this book to my late momma, Brenda Jean. I cannot put into words the amount of love, support and silliness you have instilled in me as a mother. I truly appreciate how you made motherhood look so easy while battling your own demons. I love and miss you dearly and hope this book makes you proud.

Introduction

If you have picked up this guide, you may be wondering if something like this is right for YOU...*can a little book like this really help me be more JOYful?* I cannot say this book is for everyone. I do, however, feel that this book, these stories, these tools, and these resources can help a majority of mothers, like you. Whether it be before conception or years after having a child, there may be something in this book that can help. In reality, the process of becoming a mother changes who and what you are, and it sometimes takes work, education, mindfulness, and reflection to figure out what that looks like, exactly. My goal is to help uncover that joy along your journey, to harness and manifest the life of happiness you fully deserve, and to do so in a timely manner; because let's be honest here, mommas, we don't have the time to be reading a self-help novel. If you can take just one thing from this book, put it into practice, and make a positive change toward self-improvement in your life, I will be fulfilled as an author.

This book is for those that are:

- Thinking about becoming pregnant and wondering what kind of mother they will be
- On their fertility journey
- Currently pregnant, and thus are technically already a mother
- Just bringing their baby home for the first time, full of joy and worry
- Feeling stuck in the depths of new motherhood
- Not quite as "motherly" as the lady next door
- Years into being a mother, and still feeling stuck
- A second-time mother, not feeling the same this time around
- Mothers seeking positive transformation through self-improvement
- Like-minded wellness facilitators striving to help others

CHAPTER I

My Story

Without going into too much detail and bogging you down with a long-winded story that isn't yours, I do still feel the importance of giving you my background to shed some light on what got me to this moment. Your journey will not be the same as mine; they are all so unique, and that is okay. But reading other people's stories, and speaking to other like-minded mothers, has always given me a little more peace inside — a little more confidence. Just knowing that I was not alone in the feelings I had gave me the drive to keep moving forward towards finding MY joy again. I hope this can do the same for you.

I believe my conditioning on being a mother began when I was a small child. As most subconscious conditioning is ingrained before the age of seven and solidified by fourteen, I noticed at an early age that I wasn't necessarily a "motherly" female. I didn't take to caring for dolls. I didn't want to hold small babies. Sports and being competitive were what made me happy. Most of my friends were boys. I didn't like to babysit. I tried babysitting a four-year-old boy when I was a preteen, and I absolutely hated it. It was the longest three hours of my life. Couldn't pay me enough money. I never did it again. At that very moment, the doubt started creeping into my head about being able to care for my own children in the future, without even knowing it.

Would I ever like to be around children? Is it normal to not want to babysit when a lot of my girlfriends were doing it and loving it? Is it normal that I would rather play sports with the boys? Blah, blah, blah! (We will get into that negative self-talk and how it can be so detrimental later in the book.)

Fast forward ten years: After graduating college on a full athletic scholarship, I was now a competitive beach volleyball player, traveling the Midwest and East Coast, striving to make a living doing what I loved. Not a worry in the world. Or was there? Female friends and acquaintances all around me were getting married, getting pregnant, and starting to have families. They were onto the next chapter of their lives while I was still riding that wave of being a competitive athlete.

Why do I feel so far apart from them? Why isn't starting a family on MY mind? Will I even want children?

Mentally I was nowhere close, and so the conditioning continued. I was at the start of my independent beach volleyball career, and a majority of the women I knew were moving in a totally different direction in life.

A couple of years later, I married a like-minded athlete that supported my journey. For years we traveled together, competing, submerging ourselves in that carefree, independent lifestyle. It's during that time that I decided to become a personal trainer and yoga instructor. I knew I wanted to be in the wellness space for a living. Abandoning my bachelors degree in Computer Science, I got certified in as many training programs as possible and gained as much knowledge as I could to help people lead healthier lifestyles. Not only could I help others, which I know now is my soul's purpose, but I could STILL lead that spirited lifestyle, play volleyball, and be free. I could make my own schedule and support my volleyball career. Win-win, right? I was one of the lucky ones, right? Yes, I look back and feel extremely grateful for what I was able to do but was unaware of the subconscious toll it was taking on me.

My close friends were getting pregnant with their second babies...why is there STILL no desire in ME to have a baby?

At this point I was 30. The clock was a-tickin', but I was in another time zone. My husband and I continued our journey, but it was becoming very apparent that it was much more of a friendship than an intimate marriage. We were great roommates, had so much fun together, were very like-minded in our thinking and values, but had no spark for intimacy. None. At that point, almost ten years of my life had gone by spending time with someone that I knew would never be in a position to start a family with me. Ten years of telling myself:

Maybe I wasn't born to have a child. Maybe it's not in the cards for me. Do I actually want a child? How can I have a child with no intimacy? I can be happy without a child, right?

Man do I wish I had the tools back then that I have now! The amount of junk in the back of my head that had accumulated needed an outlet. Something had to change, because deep down, in my gut (not my head), I knew I felt differently. The relationship that I had with my first husband, though wonderful in so many ways, was ten years of more of the same conditioning. You cannot have a child without intimacy, so I convinced myself that I was never going to be a mother, and that was how it was *supposed* to be.

During the next few years, I threw myself into my new career. I took a break from athletics and training and got into the medical device industry. I put everything I had into growing a nonexistent territory into a two-million-dollar sales business. I became the breadwinner in our marriage and was financially independent. I called my own shots and had full control over my life. It was time. I could take care of myself.

As my first husband and I parted ways (*maybe I did want to be a mom after all?*), my plan was to roll with what life brought to me. Take life day by day, find peace and happiness in myself, see what the world had in store for me. Eat healthy. Do yoga. Start meditating. That is exactly what I did. The last thing I had on my mind was getting into another relationship. I was 34 years old at this point, had come to a peaceful place in my life, was successful and felt in control. But something was still missing.

Then bam!! Enter my second husband. An extremely handsome and fun-loving younger man who had a huge family, loved children, and was the poster child for intimacy. Couldn't keep his hands off of me. Funny how the universe works, huh? Amazing how finding love becomes so easy once you truly love yourself. I couldn't deny the chemistry and fun that we had and truly felt that this was where I was supposed to be. Within two years, I was married and discussing the possibility of starting a family. One year later, after just one week of getting off of birth control, I was pregnant. Yes, pregnant. Say what?! Hold the damn phone.

It usually takes at least six months to get pregnant after birth control, right? How did it happen so quickly? Is my body telling me something? Can I handle being pregnant? What did I just do?

Now let's think about this. Just two short years before, I had come to terms with the fact that I may be that 40-year-old lady (no cats though), single, contemplating the option of adopting a child. I had a busy career and called my own shots. Mentally I was extremely far away from the thought of having a child. In addition, all of that past conditioning had me convinced that I would probably never have a child of my own. Now I was one week sans birth control pill and the pregnancy test said positive. Deep breaths, people. Deep breaths.

I was terrified.

(I want to mention here that looking back now, I am full of gratitude for becoming pregnant so quickly. I have worked with, and am friends with, so many women who struggle to become pregnant. My goal is not to be unappreciative of the ability to get pregnant quickly, but to further demonstrate how MY journey has conditioned my subconscious.)

It was at this point in my life, I believe the conditioning slowed, but the doubt started taking over because of that conditioning. Beliefs manifest into reality (Repeat: Beliefs Manifest into Reality), and my conditioned negative beliefs were starting to creep into my reality.

Am I going to be a good mother? Am I too old for this? What the hell did I get myself into?

To be honest I was now even more terrified.

But wasn't I supposed to be excited and full of joy?

Other than the normal aches and pains, nausea in my first trimester, and a handful of reality checks when it came to what I could and couldn't do (drink wine), I had a fairly easy and healthy pregnancy. Did I enjoy being pregnant? Absolutely not. Not for one second. It was probably the longest nine months of my life, to be honest. But with that being said, I continued to be grateful and thankful that I was having a healthy pregnancy and was able to carry a baby so well for being considered "advanced age" in the medical community (another topic that negatively plays with your subconscious).

Enter the one-and-only Birth Plan. Oh, the birth plan! I believe this should be called the "You really don't have any control over what is going to happen, so you better be able to roll with the punches, plan." My birth plan did nothing other than set me up for mental failure. It also contributed to the negative self-talk that took place all throughout my pregnancy.

Can I do this naturally? Should I give birth at a hospital or a birthing center? What if I want meds? What if I have to be induced? What if I need a C-section? Does the medical community have my best interests in mind?

These were all things I didn't have much control over at all. I went through delivery in a totally different manner than planned and it took yet another toll on the conditioned mind that I was already battling.

The real struggle for me started when I held my son for the first time. It is extremely hard to admit, but I wasn't one of those mothers who had that instant connection with her child when they were put on her chest (go figure). I was exhausted! All I wanted to do was sleep. I knew I loved him and was definitely proud of what we had all just accomplished, but I was overwhelmed and in shock.

What did I just get myself into? Can I handle this?

Although there were so many times of happiness, laughter, and joy, everything was slightly overshadowed by this grey cloud that followed me. Breastfeeding was extremely difficult for me and only lasted one month (my plan had been to make it to six). My son had a very strong Moro reflex, which meant it was very difficult to get him down to sleep, and he almost never stopped moving. I don't operate well tired (more on being a Human Design Projector later in the book), so you can imagine the first three months. I deal with chronic neck and back pain from years of sports and injuries, so physically it took a significant toll on my 37-year-old body. I don't mention these things to complain or dwell, but to reassure you that you are not alone if you too feel some of these things. These are all very common pieces to the puzzle of new motherhood, but it doesn't downplay the fact that the struggle is real, and finding tools, resources, and support is extremely important. It may be the most important thing you can do as a new mother.

Over the next few years, as I grew as a mother, becoming entrenched in self-improvement, pre- and post-natal health, energy-based wellness, and working with hundreds of clients, I realized I needed to write this book. Motherhood completely changed who I am today, and without these tools, I'm not quite sure where I would be. Everything I had experienced and had been conditioned to think in the past snowballed into years of mental combat. I didn't personally see the light and joy in being a mother until my son was three years old. Truth. My goal is to help you manifest your joy sooner. As I move through the following chapters, I hope you can take bits and pieces and apply it where necessary. Making just small changes in different facets of your life can make a world of difference, and you are completely worthy of all the joy and happiness available. Mothers are rock stars, in my opinion, and truly are my heroes.

CHAPTER 2

Why Do I Feel Like an Alien?

HORMONAL CHANGES

Oh, hormones. Progesterone, Estrogen, Relaxin, hCG, hPL...the list goes on. In all reality, they are the common denominator for all things "alien" that happen to our body and mind during our journeys. Whether it be the hormones injected during fertility treatments, the hormones created during pregnancy, or the ones we face postpartum, they are definitely the simple answer to the question "Why do I feel like an alien?" More specifically, the necessary hormones that allow us to fertilize an egg, grow an additional organ, nourish a fetus, pump 50 percent more blood within our bodies, loosen and open our bodies for delivery, prepare our breasts for feeding, and allow our bodies to recover, like anything, come with negative side effects. And it's only in our later years, after we have children, that we start to dig deeper into how these deficiencies or surpluses can negatively affect us. I definitely see a need for earlier exploration and detection in this field from a medical and holistic standpoint. Not only does this potentially wreak permanent havoc on our physical bodies in terms of weight gain, increased foot size, bladder incontinence, vaginal widening, saggy breasts, and stretch marks; more importantly, it can have a serious negative impact on the mind. Mood swings, fatigue, anxiety, and depression are all directly linked to estrogen and progesterone levels in the body. Combine that with any past conditioned negative thoughts, exhaustion, and a crying baby, and you have a recipe for potential disaster.

BODY CHANGES

Aside from all of the wonderful things that are happening inside our bodies that we can't actually see, the obvious body changes can also take a toll on how we perceive ourselves as new mothers. From vaginal damage, to C-section scars, stretch marks, hair loss, diastasis of the abdominal muscles, irregular breasts, and constant puffiness, it's no wonder that we can easily fall into a negative mind space. Was breastfeeding a breeze? Are you able to recover and rest as much as you need? Can you work out right now to get your body back? Do you feel like the supermom you were hoping for? No, No, No, and No. Although these are also the things that can make us tough and proud and resilient, it's absolutely common and normal to struggle with these changes. How could we not? In a time when we as mothers are supposed to be so happy and eternally grateful for this new life, it's imperative that we take the time to recognize the signs of mental illness and take the time and energy to work on our self-improvement journey to joy, even if its minimal. The mental health of a new mother is directly related to the mental health of those around her. Since suicide has been found to be one of the leading causes of death in new mothers (what a nauseating statistic), it's time to start addressing the red flags and stop ignoring the signs. It's okay. It's common. You are not alone. There is hope, support, and resolution.

But where do we start?

CHAPTER 3

Rewiring the Mind

THE JOURNEY

By definition, *journey* means the act of traveling from one place to another. Seems pretty cut and dried, right? Not in my opinion. A journey is taking one moment at a time, being mindful of that moment, and trusting that you are exactly where you need to be. It's not so much tangible, like going from point A to point B with a final destination, but an ever-moving and changing wave that you have to learn to ride — a wave that never really comes to shore. We first must realize and trust that we have our own story, are so very beautifully unique, and must pioneer our own journey back to JOY.

"Trust that you soul has a plan, and even if you can't see it completely, know that everything will unfold as it is meant to."
– Deepak Chopra

I believe it takes a lot of practice and self-reflection to come to terms with the fact that everything around us is happening for a reason and is a part of our wave-like journey. That reason is unique to YOU, your environment, your body, your spirituality, your family, your life. It all takes time. Fertility, or lack thereof, has a way of testing that journey; and it's during this phase of life where we can lose faith, our beliefs, our spirituality, or whatever it may be that guides us. Our goal here is to acknowledge that our journeys are beautifully unique and ultimately meant to be. Our guides are always there, right by our side and available for support. There will be ups and downs, but we can come through on the other side, more enlightened, freer, and more joyful.

I believe the next two sections of this book (PSYCH-K and Human Design) are the most important pieces to the puzzle with regard to knowing why you are here on this earth, hence becoming closer to joy. Becoming in-tune with our soul's purpose is the goal here. In that knowing, you can successfully manifest joy from the right energy space and with the right tools. It's in this research and experimenting where we can clear out the bad to make more room for the good. Where we truly get in touch with our inner knowing. Simply put, let us clear the subconscious cobwebs with PSYCH-K to allow for your unique Human Design energy blueprint to lead you to JOY.

PSYCH-K

As I mentioned earlier in the book, most of our programming is fully engrained by the time we are seven years of age (some research suggests fourteen), including the good, the bad, and the ugly. We can absolutely be negatively conditioned later in life through society, culture, family, the environment, trauma, and loss, but that fragile first seven years of our life really tells our brain subconsciously how to act, react, and think as we move through our conscious flow. Those nuggets have great power over our perceived reality and how we move through our daily lives in the now. Think of it like an iceberg with 10 percent of it being exposed and the other 90 percent below the surface. The small tip above water represents the conscious mind, the thoughts you are aware of every day, and the lower part underneath the water, the subconscious. The subconscious cannot be seen but takes up a majority of the iceberg and also takes up a majority of our perception and action. Unfortunately, we don't know how some of those limiting beliefs and conditioning are affecting us until we dive deeper into our modern-day struggles. Enter motherhood.

Modern-day psychologists and wellness facilitators use several techniques to address the subconscious (or the unconscious, as it is also called), including but not limited to meditation, hypnosis, soul reprogramming, brain entrainment device treatments, traditional talk therapy, and PSYCH-K. Although I believe all of these techniques are viable options, worth exploring, and are unique to each person, I want to discuss PSYCH-K a bit more because that is what truly worked for me. In addition, I think it is a very straightforward and simple process that can be done in a timely manner. It doesn't require multiple sessions of talk therapy and can even be done virtually. My goal in seeking therapy for the subconscious was to dig deeper into some of my anxiety (past fears) and postpartum depression (limiting beliefs manifesting from those fears) to open space for more joy. I felt that I could read hundreds of self-help books and meditate until the cows come home, but until I addressed what was stuck in my subconscious, I would just be spinning my wheels. I could want to change something so badly, but if that 90 percent of my brain below the surface wasn't playing along, it was a lost cause. I am so glad I did. It changed my life. It allowed me to shed the necessary negative layers to my mind that were holding me back from finding who I was really supposed to be on this planet.

In a nutshell, PSYCH-K is a psychological and scientific process designed to rewire subconscious programming for self-improvement. Based on neuroscience, quantum science, and brain dominance theory, it also brings the mind/body/soul connection into the fold. I like to think of myself as having a science-based energy-driven spirituality, so this was right up my alley: scientific backing with an element of personal spirituality thrown in (whatever that may look like for you). The process is performed through verbally and physically balancing the two brain hemispheres by proven muscle testing and providing transformative positive statements to rewire the limiting beliefs. First recalling situations in your life, though potentially seemingly insignificant, that can have a huge negative impact on the brain. For example, I had a traumatic event happen to me when I was 12 years old. Houses in my neighborhood were getting burglarized left and right, and I remember lying in my bed many nights, terrified that it was going to happen to us. Well, it did. Not only did we get burglarized, but our house was burnt down in the process. We also lost our dog. Although a hugely traumatic event in hindsight, in the moment I had no clue how it would affect me as an adult. I realized through PSYCH-K therapy that this event implanted deep seated fear into my brain, stuck for years without being addressed, manifesting into major fear-based anxiety today. After uncovering the trauma, muscle testing how to properly address that fear, I was able to balance the statement in my brain of "I am safe, and the universe has my back" until that limiting belief was gone. A muscle test to confirm was performed. It was very simple, to the point and very effective. Another example was an event I had in college. After a long day of volleyball practice my whole team got stuck in the elevator on the way up to our locker room. The doors would not open, and it was continually going back and forth from the first and second floors. After about 20 minutes of messing with the buttons, it finally opened and all 13 of us poured out. Again, although somewhat funny and insignificant at the time, I believe that is what kickstarted my need to be in control, which in turn led to me having panic attacks while flying. My subconscious brain correlated the two. After testing and performing the necessary PSYCH-K balances, I was able to retrain my brain to think and know that "I am safe going with the flow". Over the course of a few months and five PSYCH-K sessions, as I was peeling the layers back and discovering more negative subconscious beliefs, I was able to address and balance more than ten limiting beliefs that were holding me back. Each time I left my session I felt lighter (even dizzy sometimes), less burdened, extremely relieved, liberated, and more open to the joy that was being sent to me from the universe. The universe and our gods are here to help and guide us, but we first must re-wire and make the space. I highly recommend seeking out a licensed PSYCH-K facilitator. It will absolutely be worth your time and... well, energy!

Recommended Virtual Facilitator: Elli Richter (@ ellirichter)

HUMAN DESIGN

Speaking of energy, 'The Human Design Experiment', as some call it, has to be the most important and most interesting portion of this book, in my opinion. It has singlehandedly changed the way I view myself, how I make decisions, how I parent, how I work, how I love, how I think, and how I move through this universe from an energy standpoint on a daily basis. It has also taught me how to better interact with my spouse and son, and to me that is priceless. It made so much of an impact on me that just three short weeks after being introduced to it through my PSYCH-K sessions, I began the journey of becoming certified in facilitating BodyGraph charts to help spread the word among my clients, family, and friends. Human Design is a huge part of my wellness business to this day. It has allowed me to be okay, and increasingly more joyful, with who I actually am and am meant to be. Experimenting with Human Design can be very transformational; validating our place in this world, empowering our knowledge of our universal makeup, liberating us from societal pressures, providing peace of mind about our uniqueness, and trusting the steps and actions we take on this planet. Once we can begin to fully understand our unique one-of-a-kind energy blueprint, we drop the chatter that weighs us down and open up space to live the life we were designed to live. As both human beings and mothers. That, to me, is true JOY.

As for some history, Human Design was developed in 1987 by a gentleman by the name of Alan Robert Krakower. After earning a Bachelor of Arts degree, his career path led him into the business world as an advertising executive, magazine publisher, and media producer. In 1983, he left Canada to travel, eventually finding his way to the island of Ibiza, where he spent years working as a teacher. In January 1987, he had an unusual mystical experience followed by an encounter with "The Voice," an intelligence far superior to anything he had ever experienced. This grueling, almost deadly encounter lasted for eight days and nights, during which he received a transmission of information that he called the "Human Design System." In 1989, after his encounter with The Voice, Ra Uru Hu (the name he took after the experience) wrote the Rave I'Ching, the foundation upon which Human Design rests and the key to unlocking the code of our genetics. The oldest of the Chinese classic texts, the I'Ching, or Book of Changes, is an ancient divination tool used for over three thousand years. Ra Uru Hu dedicated the next 25 years of his life to the development and teaching of the Human Design System around the world. The System combines the principles of Genetics, the I Ching, Astrology, Kabbalah, Hindu-Brahmin Chakra System, and Quantum Physics. Your chart, or BodyGraph, is generated and calculated using your birthplace, exact birth time, and date, and is a very complex look into your one-of-a-kind design.

An important note from the founder:

"The Human Design System is not a belief system. It does not require that you believe in anything. It is not stories. It is not philosophy. It is a concrete map of the nature of being. It is a logical way to see ourselves.

With Human Design, just knowing the simple mechanics of your Design isn't enough to make a vast difference in your life. The irony of what it is to be a human being is that we are caught at the surface of understanding and accepting our nature in the cosmos around us. We are just at the surface. It doesn't matter how intelligent we are. It doesn't matter the labels that we attach to that intelligence – whether we call it 'enlightened' or whether we call it 'genius'. There is a vast underlying ignorance of how our bodies operate.

The Human Design System is a reading of your genetic code. This ability to be able to detail the mechanics of your nature in such depth is obviously profound because it reveals your entire character – conscious and unconscious – in all its subtleties. However, it is not necessary for you to know human design and great depth. That is the job of the professional analyst. What this work aspires to communicate is simply the surface mechanics of your nature. This will give you grounding in your life which will immediately bring a difference to your life process.

These essential truths are simple because they are mechanical. The way in which your genes operate is purely mechanical, and the moment you try to interfere with their operation you descend into a life of confusion, chaos comma and pain. In the end, your genes will have their way.

You are passengers in these bodies. You are passenger consciousness experiencing life going by. Buddha taught that the body is not yours. It is not. Yet at the same time, you are totally dependent on it. This is the tragedy of a sick body. You are totally dependent on your vehicles. To learn how to operate them properly immediately brings benefits.

In my teaching of human design and the training of human design analysts, students of mine have range from 14 years old to being in their late 80s. There is no limitation and there is no barrier denying anyone from grasping these essential truths about themselves. This is not simply about saying "Aha, I'm this or I'm that". This is not just another profiling system. It is about having the opportunity to do something with the knowledge. It is about being able to act on it and experiment with its logic. This brings the remarkable experience of finding and ultimately living one's true life.

All learning, that is real learning, takes seven years. It takes approximately seven years to regenerate the cells in the body. We live in a seven-year cycle. The moment that you begin to come to your own nature, the moment that you allow your body to live its life without resistance, you begin a deep process of deconditioning. Years later, you emerge, quite literally, as a new being – yourself.

It's one of the great cosmic jokes that human beings don't have the opportunity to live out their own lives. It is because they don't have the opportunity to live out their own lives that life seems to be such a difficult experience for them. We know that there is a lot of rhetoric around being yourself. It is all fine and good for somebody to stand up and tell you to be yourself, but first you have to know who that self is.

In my professional work, I have given thousands of readings. Wherever that has been, and regardless of culture or country, I have found there to be one prevailing disease. That disease is self-hatred, and it thrives wherever you discover something about yourself that you would like to change. Self-hatred varies in intensity from being just beneath the surface of the consciousness, to being full blown. It is the most human of ironies that self-hatred is truly misplaced because most people do not know themselves. They actually hate the wrong person. They are actually dissatisfied with the wrong person.

Most human beings don't like themselves and they don't like themselves because they truly do not know who they are. Most human beings have never lived the experience of being themselves nor seen the beauty of what their true life holds. It is time to see that this is not, as the ancients claim, the planet of suffering, but in fact, an opportunity for a glorious awareness.

Human design is not about guarantees or promises. This is not saying that if you live out your own nature, you're going to be the wealthiest or the most beautiful. It is not about being better or best. It is about being yourself.

Life is a duality, and this is revealed through our moralities. There is always going to be this in that. There is always going to be the good and the bad. There is always going to be success and there is always going to be failure. That is the nature of what it is to be human.

The moment that you live out your own nature and you enter into life correctly; this is the moment that you get what is correct for you. You get the correct career, and you get the correct relationships. So, you see, it does not matter whether you are a success or not, because there will be no suffering despite your state. You will be living out your nature and it will be clear to you that what is there for you is right for you, whatever that might be. Only then, finally, will there be no part of you that can say: 'I wish I could be something else or somewhere else'.

We are overwhelmed in our western culture with improvement propaganda. The hucksters cry 'be thinner, wiser, faster and richer'. There are all kinds of purveyors of teachings who beckon us to follow their way. All human beings suffer from the propaganda of generalizations. Without knowing oneself, one can so easily be lost in this propaganda. You do not have to change anything. It is simply a matter of becoming yourself and becoming aware of yourself.

The Human Design System opens the doors to the potential of self-love. Finding self-love is about finding a greater love, a love for life and a love for others through understanding. Throughout this living your design course in seeing yourself and in coming to understand how you can live out your own nature, please pay attention to the importance of that in your relationship with others. So many of our difficulties in this life are because we have great difficulties in our relationships, whether they are our business relationships or whether they are our personal relationships.

To be yourself is to bring into your life those people who are truly for you. This knowledge is about how you do that simply, so that you too can benefit from the best possible associations. Correct associations allow you to not only be seen and understood by others, but also allow you to understand them. As a parent, this has been an essential ingredient in the well-being of my children.

Human Design is logical, mechanical knowledge. It is neither theorizing nor philosophy. It is about being able to do practical things with knowledge that brings practical benefits. I hope you enjoy living your design and that you too can participate in becoming a healthy, self-loving human being.

– Ra Uru Hu,
Living Your Design Student Manual

True joy is buried within the knowing of oneself.

Curious about your chart? So was I! It is a beautiful rabbit hole of profound information. I am so very grateful that I was introduced to this experiment. Not only did I dive in for my own health and well-being, but like I mentioned before, I have dedicated a majority of my wellness business to helping other people live their design. It's so very helpful in finding your true momma JOY. I recommend taking a minute to find out the exact minute, date, and location of your birth and plugging it in to any of the free chart generation sites or apps available right now. It's also a great idea to explore your partner's and children's charts as well.

Here is a FREE recommended app (*Human Design for Us All*) and website link (https://www.jovianarchive.com) to get you started.

Getting familiar with your energy type is the best place to start. I explain each of the five Human Design types briefly below as I truly believe this is one of the biggest leaps you can take in finding your JOY. I suggest finding your type and reading the description. This is just the first layer of understanding your chart and how it may resonate with you. It goes much much deeper if the desire to experiment is there (relationships, emotions, digestion, parenting, brain design, personality, etc). Remember, there is nothing to believe here. This is just a guide on how you are designed to move and interact in space. The explanations below will go over your type, your authority, your strategy, your signature, and your "Not Self" theme. Further layers can be peeled as you dive deeper into your design and those of your loved ones, if you are so inclined. In my opinion, it is worth every second. If everyone had more peace of mind, inner knowing, liberation, and confidence moving through this life, it would be a very harmonious one, to say the least!

To find out more about my human design service offerings, please visit www.kings-medical.com/human-design-experiment and/or follow @kings.wellness on Instagram.

GENERATORS (35% OF THE POPULATION)

Generators house the magnetic life force for all. You are here for the dance of life and to create positive energy and spark for yourself and others. Generators have the uncanny ability to truly change the world. You are THE authority in our universe and are here to lift others around you. Once you get lifted first, you lift others without any effort! You are a natural hustler with an extremely sparkly and attractive aura when living your true design.

Generators are prone to a lot of past negative conditioning because historically they were taken advantage of and used. They were praised as children for making other people happy, and that is not what truly makes a generator happy. This past conditioning created a path away from your actual design but gives you so much room to grow in this experiment. It's important here to listen to your gut and act on your own desires, not what you "should" be doing. If it's not a "Hell Yes!" then it's a "Hell No!"

To do this you must make decisions based on your **Authority, which is from the GUT**, literally. You are ruled by your sacral chakra, and your instincts and desires are extremely visceral. Asking the gut simple "yes or no" or "this or that" questions are best. The gut has no in between or storytelling capabilities. You learn best as you go, trusting that your body will lead you in the right direction to get a response. You must dance with life as it comes. You won't have all of the answers before you begin. That's okay! Think of the universe as your personal shopper. Your **strategy as a Generator is to RESPOND** to those positive messages, and DO, once you get that positive gut response. You must also be somewhat selfish in that sense and learn to say no (kindly and with respect) to things that don't serve you. Once you clear out the no's and the things that don't speak to your gut in a positive way, you create this neutral space where the universe will reward you with that life force, success, love, and positive energy. People LOVE being around generators that are true to their design. You are the spark and joy of every party in that sense and bring so much life to everyone around you!

Lastly, you will know you aren't living your design when your "not self" response kicks in. **Your Not Self response is FRUSTRATION**. Frustration in terms of pent-up emotions or in the sense of blocked energy. This is your signpost or red flag to correct your course, get rid of some of the no's to make room for the positivity. Less "doing" things to please others, more room for the universe to drop in the good. If you don't listen to that Frustration flag and don't allow that course to correct, burnout and depletion will be the result. Burnout and depletion tell you that you aren't listening to your cues from the universe. Just have faith that the universe will have your back, if you make the room for it, by clearing out the things that don't speak to you. **Your signature when truly living your design is SATISFACTION**. You will feel that "Ahhhh" feeling when you are on the right path to your design.

Famous Generators: Albert Einstein, the Dalai Lama, Elvis Presley, Bill Clinton, Meryl Streep, Madonna, George Harrison, Judy Garland, James Dean, Oprah Winfrey, Deepak Chopra, Margaret Thatcher

MANIFESTING GENERATORS (35% OF THE POPULATION)

Manifesting Generators (MGs) have the biggest engine of all human types, with a very expansive energy field. You are one of the most limitless thinkers and visionaries of our world. You are here to follow your bliss. MGs are a mix of spontaneity (M) and Bliss seeker (G). Your goal in life is to lift others up, unintentionally, by lifting yourself up and making life less linear.

MGs can't be put into a box; they are not linear. It's like putting a square peg into a circle. MGs have many passions, and those interests and passions are what bring you your joy...in turn bringing joy to those around you. It's normal for a MG to have two professions at once and to move around those passions and professions quickly, as long as they are both serving your joy. It's also important to reserve the right to change your mind often, and to also inform your family and friends that you do so with good intention.

You are ruled by your **Authority of the GUT,** like true Generators. You must pay attention to what physically and viscerally moves you. Like generators, your **strategy as a Manifesting Generator is to RESPOND** to those positive messages, and DO, once you get that positive gut response. You will know in the pit of your stomach. Don't overthink things. If you can't explain it, it's right. If your mind can explain the feeling, it's not a gut urge. You must be okay with the unknown from that point on. That is where the spontaneity and bliss come in.

It's important for you to not over-extend yourself too far in the future and to always take inventory of what is serving you and what isn't. You may find yourself excited about something initially, then when the time comes to actually go do it...you don't want to do it. Sound familiar? It's very important to alleviate some of the negativity to make more room for the positivity to drop in from the universe. If not, you will experience burnout.

Lastly, like Generators, you will know you aren't living your design when your "not self" response kicks in. **Your Not Self response is FRUSTRATION**. Frustration in terms of either pent up emotions or in the sense of blocked energy. This is your signpost or red flag to course correct, get rid of some of the no's, to make room for the positivity. Less "doing" things to please others, more room for the universe to drop in the good. If you don't listen to that Frustration flag and don't allow that course to correct, burnout and depletion will be the result. Burnout and depletion tell you that you aren't listening to your cues from the universe. Just have faith that the universe will have your back, if you make the room for it, by clearing out the things that don't speak to you. **Your signature when truly living your design is SATISFACTION.** You will feel that "Ahhhh" feeling when you are on the right path to your design.

Famous MGs: Frederic Chopin, Hillary Clinton, Clint Eastwood, Sigmund Freud, Mahatma Gandhi, Marie Antoinette, Mikhail Gorbachev, Jimi Hendrix, Pope John Paul II, Janis Joplin, Richard Nixon, Yoko Ono, Prince, Jacqueline Onassis, Martin Luther King, Vincent Van Gogh

PROJECTORS (21% OF THE POPULATION)

Projectors are here to guide, to tweak, and to bring efficiency to the systems around us. As the most complex auric type, they have the special ability to see things in ways others can't and are here to guide the tribe with their insight. Projectors are a non-energy type that doesn't initiate; they help better when being initiated. Since projectors were the last human type to arrive in 1781, they aren't made to go-go-go, and were made to better our universe. They have been conditioned to hustle and keep up with the rest of the world, but they are not here to do that. Projectors must trust the flow of life and allow themselves to rest when needed.

Projectors' **Authority comes from the Spleen,** which means quick instinct is your guide. Plain and simple. It is there to keep you alive and can be trusted fully. Every splenic feeling you honor can take you that much closer to wellbeing. You may find yourself saying often, "I just knew that was going to happen!", or "I smell a rat!", because, well, you did. Don't overthink; the mind is not designed to make decisions.

Projectors are built to "work" efficiently for only a few hours a day. It's imperative that they honor and respect their energy and use it wisely. Projectors are also absorbing beings, so they take on all of the energy of those around them and it gets magnified substantially. It is very important for projectors not only to know that the energy is not theirs, but also to release that energy often with Epsom salt baths, sage burning, alone time, rest, solo walks, etc. Projectors are here to newly define the energy field of CEOs. They can be deemed as "pushy" or "bossy" or "know it all" due to past conditioning. Projectors are served best to indulge in knowledge and learning, and to work on those things they can "do in their sleep." It's when resting that the true guidance shines through.

The Strategy of a projector is to Wait for the Invitation. Once an invitation (physical or energetically) and openness has been granted, the projector can then begin to help and guide others with their extremely intuitive and insightful knowledge. In a world trained to "Just Do It," this can be a challenge. Once this is honored, the **signature of a projector is true SUCCESS.** The justification of your design will then shine through. The best way for people to recognize you is by recognizing yourself. You don't need approval from others, but you do need that invite.

Lastly, you will know you aren't living your true design when the **Not Self of BITTERNESS** shows up. Feeling victimized or bitter about someone or something is a sign that you need to course correct. If you allow bitterness to take over, you will suffer extreme fatigue and potential illness.

Famous Projectors: Queen Elizabeth II, Mick Jagger, Joseph Stalin, Ringo Starr, Osho, Napoleon, Woody Allen, Salvador Dali, Elizabeth Taylor, Fidel Castro,

James Joyce, Barbra Streisand, Ulysses S. Grant, Douglas MacArthur, Demi Moore, Princess Diana, Tony Blair, Ramana Maharshi, George Gurdjieff

MANIFESTORS (8% OF THE POPULATION)

Manifestors are energy beings with the biggest and most selective auras. They are meant to embrace their bigness, be spontaneous, and not be put into a box. They are the only initiator type that don't have to wait for anything external to make things happen. They are true trailblazers, fire starters, and natural "Just Do It" leaders. Manifestors are meant to rally, gather, and create momentum in this universe.

It is important to **INFORM; that is the Manifestor Strategy**. Not to micromanage, plan, or strategize, just be transparent. As long as Manifestors inform others of their actions, it is coming from good, and no one will be hurt in doing so; they are free to do. Not informing will lead to much resistance and pushback. Manifestors cannot be told what to do or how to do it, but people around you will want to know what you are doing and why you are doing it. Your aura demands it. In learning to honor that, the right people will gravitate to you and hop aboard your train! You are the energetic team leader and train driver with beautiful bursts of positive energy.

Authority for Manifestors lies within. You must listen to that *urge* (out of nowhere that you can't make sense of) versus the *want* (can explain). That is when you know you are honoring your authority and true design. Cherish and honor the impulses; they are rare, special, and divine within you. You must own your own uniqueness and never listen to the "should." There will be people that don't like you or what you do; you aren't here to please everyone. You aren't an all-inclusive person and are here to trailblaze and initiate what you feel within.

Manifestors will know they are not living their true design when the **Not Self of ANGER** shows up. Suppressed anger can build up when you are not honoring your strategy and authority and is a signpost for course correction. This is the flow to live by: URGE – *Harm?* – EXPLAIN – DO – and the rest will follow. It's that simple. Manifestors may be conditioned to be put in a box or told what to do their entire childhood, or that they were "small," but in recognizing the red flags, it's quite an experiment to course correct and let the universe do what's best for you and those all around you. The Manifestor **Signature of healthy design comes in the form of Peace**. You will know you are at peace when you feel in control and powerful.

Famous Manifestors: Johnny Depp, Richard Burton, George W. Bush, Adolf Hitler, Frida Kahlo, Jack Nicholson, Robert DeNiro, Orson Welles, Susan Sarandon

REFLECTORS (1% OF THE POPULATION)

Reflectors are our most rare energy type and the only lunar beings on the planet; all other types are solar beings with inner authority. You are a non-energy being, with zero energy centers defined, meaning you are the mirror with an uncanny ability to embody the wisdom of all of those around you. Just like the moon doesn't generate its own light and reflects the light of the sun, so do reflectors mirror, absorb, and magnify the energy of others. Your natural state is cool, calm, and collected; and you have the ability to be anything and everything you want. You are the non-emotional conduit that we all need on this planet! You are truly the center of the tribe, reflecting all that is good in others, but unique in your own right.

Conditioning that you may feel from being a reflector is trouble in defining yourself. Where do I fit in? Am I seen as weak? It is important for the reflector to get out of his or her own way. You are not alone; you belong in the middle, surrounded by your environment. That "sensitivity" allows you to live your design, allows life to carry you and to harness whatever it is that you want to be from others.

The **Strategy of a Reflector is to Wait a Lunar Cycle.** Decisions are made in 28-day mini-episodes, and it is important to keep track of exactly how you are feeling and what is happening during those cycles. Journals are very helpful for this. The trick is to allow yourself to wait a month to process issues and experience the world, and if after 28 days the issue is still there, it's time to deal with it. You are very receptive to others, so it's important to put yourself in environments where you feel free and good. When emotions rise for the good, you are in the right place, exactly where you are supposed to be to receive. It's important here to resist pulling away and to take back your unique power of being a true chameleon in life. That doesn't happen overnight with reflectors.

The inner **Authority of the reflector is also lunar.** With no defined centers, it is important to discuss decisions (the Big Ones) with those closest to you before committing. This doesn't mean that you unload your problems on others, but you use them as a soundboard to mirror and reflect what will best serve you and the universe. It is important for reflectors to use the 28-day lunar cycle to really feel out their decisions. A lot can change over 28 days, and it is imperative to take that time to observe.

Because the reflector self is open, you are designed to wear many hats over your lifetime and engage in as many things that make you happy. When you are truly living your design, you will feel a **Signature theme of surprise and delight**! In these feelings your spontaneous purpose will surface. As a reflector it's important to ask yourself "Who am I going to be today?" and "What new experience will I have today?" These types of questions set you up to live your design and be open to what will be mirrored and reflected to best serve you in that moment. The **Not Self theme of a reflector is disappointment**. When you are not living your design, that signpost will tell you to course correct, possibly change environments or give yourself more time (28 days). The true nature of a reflector is to surround yourself with good vibes and curate what is best for you and your community.

Famous Reflectors: H.G. Wells, Sandra Bullock, Fyodor Dostoyevsky, Ammachi, Michael Jackson

The point here is to be at peace with who you are and to better know how to interact with the world around you; to work on ridding yourself of the things that aren't yours, and truly know what does serve you; to better communicate with yourself and with all of those around you; to be open and curious as to what authority you have within, and to support the ability to find more joy; to find liberation from what society is telling you to do and move through life as your genuine authentic self; and to harness that confidence and trust your inner knowing.

That's the good stuff, especially for a mother.

CHAPTER 4

The Importance of Mindfulness

The buzzword of the decade is Mindfulness. By definition, according to Wikipedia, mindfulness is the psychological process of purposely bringing one's attention to experiences occurring in the present moment without judgment, which one develops through the practice of meditation and through other trainings (i.e., all of things I will discuss in this chapter). There is no doubt that being mindful in your daily life takes commitment, time, and practice, but as all of the literature and studies state, it is as good as gold. Being able to train the mind to be positive, still, and in control is a superpower that we all desperately need.

But where do we start? We start with the self. We start by going inward, connecting to the source within, and creating a beautiful relationship and connection between heart, soul, body, and mind. We are all energy in this Universe, after all, and we must learn to look at and treat ourselves accordingly.

SELF-DIALOGUE AND AFFIRMATIONS

Whether our motherhood takes its form by way of adoption, in-vitro fertilization, menstrual cycle timing, scheduled intercourse, or throwing three sheets to the wind, we are all one and the same when it comes to the label of motherhood. We all have our baggage and struggles and are ultimately entering a world of unknowns. We all experience the "*should*" and/or negative self-dialogue to some degree throughout the process. The monkey mind, defined in Buddhism as "unsettled," is a very powerful force that begins to take over, telling us stories that lead us down the path of self-doubt, fear, anxiety, and depression. As I mentioned in my personal story, this happened to me the moment I got pregnant. This is where those subconscious beliefs started to create my reality. Any negative beliefs or past conditioning thoughts that are tucked away start to rear their ugly heads. This is where the shit starts to hit the fan, ladies. Most importantly, though, this is the exact moment you can start to turn things around. The sheer recognition of what's happening is all that matters. You actually have the power and control to make a positive change. The power in right now!

Recommended Read: *The Power of Now* by Eckhardt Tolle

Instead of creating a dialogue full of things that you should have done or should be doing or beating yourself up about the way things are going on your journey, now is the time to be mindful of what comes out of your mouth. Now is the time to practice changing that negative talk and those vague desires into something positive and attainable. It's now time to shift the negativity into gratitude and the ebbs and flows of the wave into appreciation. Our language plays a very important role in mental health, and how we verbalize our experiences and actions can be the difference in a positive or negative outcome.

> **"Words can inspire. And words can destroy.**
> **Choose yours well."**
> **– Robin Sharma**

But how do we practice changing that negative thought process and choosing the right language to express? As discussed earlier in the book, knowing our Human Design and working the subconscious through PSYCH-K and like-minded therapies are great starting points that allow us to clear our minds of conditioning and wipe out any preconceived notions on how we should be living our lives and mothering our children. Those tools can then set us up to being Open, Curious, Aware, Mindful, and Affirming. **Open** to the fact that you were conditioned to feel this way. **Curious** enough to want to explore change. **Aware** of the chaos that is potentially about to surface. **Mindful** of observing the change taking place. **Affirming** in how we can change the language to something more serving and positive.

One way to accomplish this is to **THINK** when it comes to self-dialogue. This simple yet effective self-check tool can be very helpful in becoming more mindful in this sense.

T – Is what I am saying 100% **T**rue?

H – Am I being **H**onest with myself?

I – What are my **I**ntentions?

N – Will this **N**egatively affect ME in any way?

K – Am I being **K**ind to myself?

Put simply, if you don't have anything nice to think, don't think it at all!

In addition, start shifting the negative self-dialogue into something more positive, serving, and intentional. For example:

Negative Self-Dialogue	Say Instead
I should....	*It's okay for me to...*
I'm never going to....	*I trust that I will....*
I can't....	*I am worthy of......*
I'm scared of.....	*It's safe for me to....*
Why am I...	*I'm right where I'm supposed to be...*
I'm not...	*I choose to...*

It is important to be respectful, loving, and truly compassionate to yourself, and to speak to yourself with true intention, as a healthy mind does not speak ill of itself or others. The more gratitude and appreciation you can give to yourself, the more you will indeed receive in return. I challenge you to start listening to that inner dialogue, making note of it, and working on ways to shift from a more negative to positive outcome. Only you can control your inner dialogue, and you may be surprised how hard we can be on ourselves.

BREATHWORK

Another crucial piece to the mindfulness puzzle is our breath; our prana as they say in yoga; our Chi, or our true life-force energy. For such an effortless function, it may be one of the most important factors in how we calm the mind, strengthen our bodies on a cellular level, and initiate movement. Not many people think about breathing on a day-to-day basis, and it takes a big shift in consciousness to learn to not only appreciate it, but to use it to our advantage. There are a few different ways that we can incorporate breathwork into our everyday lives, including specific breath-holding techniques, yogic pranayama, and mindful meditative breathing.

Working on the breath specifically as a single therapeutic healing method can be very powerful. Over the years and through multiple trainings, I've been led through a variety of different breathing techniques and ways to calm the mind, body, and spirit. Although there are differences in techniques, the common theme, in my opinion, is to connect, honor, manipulate, and cleanse: Connect to the breath as it is, being a witness to what exactly is happening. Honor that your breath is your life force and is extremely powerful in obtaining positive outcomes for mind and body wellness. Manipulate the breath in ways that calm the nervous system, create energy, still the mind, and release blocks that are holding you back. And finally, allow the breath to move through you to cleanse what needs cleansing.

One of my favorite and well known breathwork facilitators for overall health is: Wim Hoff (https://www.wimhofmethod.com/).

ENERGY WORK

I think it is also important to mention the importance of overall energy bodywork. Whether that be through massage, Reiki, tapping, or other forms of connection, it is something to consider. It goes hand in hand with breathwork and brings more awareness around the overall energy within our bodies. Once we become more educated and connected, we can then learn to harness the good and release the bad. We can learn to let go of past traumas while building fuel centers that will actually serve us. We can move the stagnation within us so our energy can flow optimally. We are all just energy moving through space, are we not? The three techniques listed below are all practices that have benefited me on my energy healing journey.

DR. JOHN AMARAL ENERGY/BODYWORK

The work I did here primarily focused on how to become aware of different energy centers within the body for the purpose of connection. Different parts of the body contain different types of energy, and through mental connection, mindfulness, meditation, visceral sounds, and breathwork, they harness a great deal of healing power. John Amaral gained notoriety on Gwyneth Paltrow's Goop Netflix series and has been pioneering energy bodywork since.

TAPPING

Tapping was another technique I used for connection. Through physical contact on different pressure points on the body, along with a rhythmic meditation, it allows for self-healing physical touch. It removes your monkey mind from the equation and gives the mind space and freedom to heal through a meditative, rhythmic feeling. Similar to snapping a rubber band on your wrist while having anxiety, this is one of the quicker methods to mind diversion. The brain has to focus on something in the now rather than the anxious or depressive thought. My favorite app for tapping is 'The Tapping Solution'.

REIKI

Probably the most profound energy bodywork I have practiced to date is Reiki. By definition, Reiki is a Japanese form of alternative medicine called energy healing. Reiki practitioners use a technique called palm healing or hands-on healing through which a "universal energy" is said to be transferred through the palms of the practitioner to the patient in order to encourage emotional or physical healing. It requires a qualified and trained Reiki master to conduct energy healing on the body. While you are laying down, calm, with eyes closed, the practitioner will move their hands slowly over the body, connecting with different energy centers, harnessing or releasing what needs to be addressed. This is where pain can be alleviated, past traumas can surface and be released, blockages can be identified, and healing can be manifested. Pain and suffering can easily reside and be stuck in the body, and Reiki is a soothing way to address that. An added bonus is possible energy connection to the other side... but we will save that topic for another book.

MEDITATION

As we learn to shift into a more positive and self-affirming dialogue with a better sense of our energy, breath, and body, it is important to know that meditation is something that can tie all of those things together in a beautiful bow. By definition (and it is truly not an easy thing to define), meditation is a practice where an individual uses a technique – such as mindfulness, or focusing the mind on a particular object, thought, or activity – to train attention and awareness and achieve a mentally clear and emotionally calm and stable state.

I believe that meditation is much simpler than that. There are no rules and there isn't a right or wrong way to do it. To me, meditation is simply having the ability to sit with your thoughts (your racing, most of the time fictional, monkey mind thoughts). It is a completely unique experience to you! It doesn't have to take hours, there doesn't have to be some big epiphany or connection with source, it may or may not include breathwork, and most importantly, it looks different for everyone. And that is okay! The important factor to remember about meditation is that you are doing it. Period. You are taking the time to check in with your thoughts. Does breathwork help you get there? Absolutely. Do certain techniques help you calm the mind so you can be a true observer? Hell yes. All of those wonderful things help and are readily available. But don't let meditation intimidate you. It is an ever-growing, progressive practice that can change your life and is worth exploring.

Below I outline a simple five-step process and sample meditation to get you started. This is something I recommend doing in bed for ten or so minutes before you reach for that phone or get up to get coffee. That timing doesn't work for you? No worries. Try it at night before bed. I have learned through my human design that I personally work best with a routine for these types of therapies, so I've created this meditation flow to make things easy, efficient, and effective.

STEP 1: CONNECTION

Connection in meditation refers to the mind/body relationship: the connection to earth and the connection to breath. Feeling your body on the bed, for example, and paying close attention to what the breath is doing at that moment. All of these connections are important when beginning your practice. Through these pathways you can become more present, less stimulated by your environment, and more in tune with your mind, body, and spirit. You will find that most meditation practices begin with some type of grounding connection to put you in the right frame of mind. These connections are also important to come back to through all stages of your meditation. Notice your mind wandering? (It absolutely will, my friend.) Allow this to bring you back to the present. This is where you allow your *conscious* mind to bring you closer to the *subconscious* work of meditation.

STEP 2: GRATITUDE

Gratitude is simply defined as the quality of reflecting and being thankful. Not only do we need to learn to be gentle and kind to ourselves, but the more we can practice being grateful for ourselves, our lives, and those people and things around us, the more the mind and our lives will flourish. In my opinion, like changing the self-dialogue from negative to positive, being grateful takes practice. It's not something that comes naturally in everyday busy life and is a learned practice and behavior. You have to make a conscious effort to pause, reflect, and verbalize gratitude, just as you do with your language. But by doing so, we speak to the universe in ways that it will listen to, appreciate, and reciprocate. Bringing gratitude into your mediation practice sets the tone for a positive experience. It allows you to privately acknowledge the things that matter in your life at that moment: thirty seconds of your time to profoundly impact the future.

STEP 3: HIGHER POWER

Opening up the channels to a higher power during meditation is a very powerful way to receive information or insight that may be helpful to you in some way. Allowing the mind to expand into the bigger picture allows for a deeper level of healing and joy. A higher power can mean different things to different people. Do you pray to God? Do you connect with Spirit? Is the Universe something that speaks to you? Maybe Buddha, Jesus, or your angels? Remember this is your mediation, your journey, and it is truly unique to you. The important thing to know here is that we have help. There is energy all around us, guiding us closer to our joy. Tapping into that energy and connecting to our higher power during mediation will get us that much closer to our inner knowing.

STEP 4: ASK FOR HEALING

Once you open up the channels to your higher power, it's time to call to action. Your higher power is listening and wants to help. Now is the time to ask for the healing that you need. Be specific with your needs and thorough with your requests. Are you battling a health issue? Ask your higher power for the healing power to remedy the situation. Are you having relationship issues? Ask for the answers. Have a very in-depth conversation with your energy and be open to receiving the response. That may come in the form of images, sounds, words, a feeling in the body, or an inner knowing. You have more control than you think over the things that you need...but you must ask and be willing to listen and accept the answer.

Now that you have been on the receiving end of the requests, it's time to share the love. This is a great time to ask your higher power to help others. Ask them to spread love, light, health, and happiness to everyone around you. Allow yourself to be the beacon that shines the light of Joy to those that surround you. Bottle up that healing magic that has been created and be a magnet for others to receive.

STEP 5: EMOTION AND VIBRATION

This last step is all about the feels. It is about bringing the meditation practice into the body and manifesting a sensation that can be taken into the rest of the day (or night). Its time here to think about a goal or intention you have for the day. It could be something as simple as "being happy" or as detailed as "finishing three chapters of my book." Once you have the goal in mind, tie that goal to a positive emotion. How will that goal make you feel emotionally today if accomplished? Will you be excited? Will you feel proud? Maybe joyful? Once you nail down the positive emotion, it's time to set the tone. Allow that emotion to fill every cell in your body. Envision that feeling as a vibration, pulsating and radiating out of every part of your body.

You are now that emotion. Every part of your being is now getting to experience that goal/emotion/vibration connection, creating a beautiful and positive wiring of the subconscious.

You now have the tools to become connected, be present, verbalize gratitude, connect to a higher power, give and receive healing, and create a positive vibration for the day; all in a ten-minute mediation session.

Powerful stuff! Want to try it out?

SAMPLE MEDITATION

Step 1

After getting comfortable and allowing all of the jitters to release, take a moment to still your body and slowly start scanning yourself from head to toe. At each body part, feel how you are connected to the surface below and imagine that connection reaching all of the way down to the earth. Notice how the body feels at each connection and feel the uplifting pressure of the earth beneath you. As you reach the tip of your toes, take your focus now to your breath. Notice how the breath is flowing in and out of the body, without trying to change it in any way. Notice how the belly and chest rise and fall with each breath and how the air feels flowing through the throat and nose. Continue to witness the breath without judgement as you notice it becoming slower and more peaceful. As the mind starts to wander throughout this mediation, always know that you can come back to the connection of body and breath. It is a powerful way to bring you back to the stillness of the present and is always available to you.

Step 2

As you continue to breathe and feel your body connected to the surfaces below, begin to think about what you are grateful for. As you think of them, silently or verbally state what you are grateful for. Take as much time as you need to acknowledge everything that comes up at that moment. If and when the mind starts to wander, come back to the body, come back to the breath, and get back to the gratitude portion of the practice. When finished, smile knowing that you have a lot to be thankful for.

Step 3

As you continue to breathe and be present, allowing your busy thoughts to come and go without attachment, start connecting to your higher power. Ask your spirit, God, Universe, whoever that may be, to open the lines of communication. Imagine floating in the cosmos, getting closer to that higher power with each breath. Thank your higher power for everything they can and will provide and know that they are always available and present.

Step 4

Now that you have opened the channels of communication, ask your higher power for healing. Ask them for any help you may need along your journey and at the present moment. Be specific in how they can help and allow their healing power to wash over your entire body like a river. Feel the energy healing in every cell of your body. Breathe in that feeling for a few moments as you allow the journey to unfold. As you continue to breathe, ask for that healing to be sent outwards to those around you. Allow the healing power to illuminate your body in a bright white ball of light, pulsating around you in every direction, touching everyone it contacts. Radiate the love that you are feeling as you continue to connect and breathe.

Step 5

Lastly, as you sit or lie there relaxed, present, and glowing, think of a goal or intention you have for the day. It can be as small or grand as you would like but hold that goal in your mind's eye.

Now think about how that goal would make you feel as you accomplish it. Bring a true emotion into the mind and body. As you pinpoint that emotion, imagine how that emotion will make you feel. Feel the vibration of that emotion throughout every cell of your body as it begins to make you feel lighter and more joyful. Continue to breathe as you allow that vibration to manifest in your subconscious and create the perfect day. For the last couple moments, let everything go and come back to the body. Scan from head to toe, feeling the connection and noting any differences this time around. Notice any feelings without judgement and let go of anything that isn't serving you. As you take a deep breath into the nose, open the mouth and let a huge sigh out. Open your eyes. Let it soak in. Be present.

Congratulations! You just meditated and you are now a Rockstar.

Please feel free to visit www.kings-medical.com/meditation for a free downloadable audio momma meditation pack.

Favorite Meditation App: Headspace

JOURNALING

Now that you've learned the tools and tricks of mindfulness, breathwork, and meditation, try journaling. A good old pen and paper is a way to really put the rubber to the road. It is a powerful tool. I repeat, it is a simple, yet powerful tool. Keeping a journal that speaks to you (and that you can speak to) can change your life. It absolutely changed mine. Again, there are no rules! Self-improvement and joy seeking are your experience alone, so customize it to your liking. It's just a matter of having a journal and your favorite pen available at all times and allowing the thoughts (positive or negative) to have an outlet. That could mean scribbling, making lists, writing paragraphs, burning statements that don't serve you (that's a fun one), taking notes, creating a morning routine, the list goes on. Keep your journal as handy as you keep your phone. Deepak Chopra commented that journaling allows you to get the junk out of your head and to move on. He was absolutely right. Not only can you release any negative thoughts, but you can then turn those thoughts and feelings into gratitude. Every situation has a silver lining and finding those slivers of gratitude will help change the thought process into something more positive, serving, and productive.

Exercise: Grab a pen and a piece of paper...yes, right now, love.

- Write down three goals for your life right now. Be vague. Be specific. Just be genuine. Take two minutes or take ten. You do you.

- With each of those, write down an emotion that speaks to that goal when accomplished (sound familiar?). Will that goal make you happy? Fulfilled? Excited? Successful? Write it ALL down.

- Last, connect with and write down a vibration or feeling in the body that the emotion will make you feel. Where will you feel that in the body? How does that look? Scribble, be organized, draw pictures. Whatever is speaking to you at this very moment. Just write it ALL down. Get it out of the mind and onto paper. Manifest it.

- Now close your eyes and visualize those feelings. Feel them in every fiber of your being. Imagine that to be your reality.

Through journaling, you have just successfully started to clear and train the mind for your self-fulfilling prophecy. Again, your thoughts manifest your reality, so start taking control of your own destiny at this very moment. Such a simple and easy tool with such a profound impact on your mental health and JOY.

CHAPTER 5

Using Nature for Healing

SUPPLEMENTATION

I truly believe that adding supplements to my daily routine helped save me. It was one of the first tangible steps I could take towards feeling better on a daily basis. Being a researcher is part of my design, so I gathered as much information as I could on my symptoms (fatigue, heart palpitations, UTIs, sweating, moodiness, weight gain, increased blood pressure, etc.) and went to town. Literally. I got the opinions of functional medical doctors, holistic life coaches, chiropractors, primary care physicians, Reiki masters and like-minded mothers to come up with a few solid supplements that would be both feasible and affordable. And it worked. Most importantly, I was making an effort. Mentally that can go a long way, ladies. The placebo effect is real. I was taking some control of my health (something I felt had been long gone) and was doing the work. I also bought a juicer, something that I had wanted for a long time but never wanted to spend the money on. I'm a frugal one! Now was the time.

I never said that finding your joy was going to be a walk in the park, but boy is it worth it. A daily smoothie concoction and healthy coffee substitution (caffeine triggers my anxiety) and fresh juice can go a long way for mental and physical health. It sets your body and mind up for success and gives you focus. If you are starting to see a theme here, it is all about self-care. We cannot care for or love other people to the fullest without loving ourselves. We cannot teach our children to honor their well-being if we don't honor our own. It is okay to be selfish in this sense. Please be. Society tells us differently, but that is where self-awareness and conditioning come in. Stop listening to what others are saying and be unapologetically you. Love yourself unconditionally first so you can love others unconditionally.

Here is what worked for me. Remember, we are all unique and all have our own set of symptoms. Please honor yourself in that sense and do what works for you, your health, and your budget. I am no medical doctor, just an educated, holistic momma who was driven to find her JOY again.

SMOOTHIE BASE

Vanilla Oat Milk (or alternative milk of choice)

Frozen Blueberries (or fruit of choice)

Raw Peanut Butter (vegan protein)

Raw Honey (healthy sweetness)

Banana (thickness/calming)

SUPPLEMENTS

These can be put into your smoothie or taken separately. I loathe pills and have a wicked gag reflex, so I break my capsules up into my smoothies for a one-two punch.

Greens Powder with Probiotics (so much goodness)

DIM Plus Natural Based Capsules (estrogen balancing/mood/fatigue)

Cranberry Capsules (healthy urinary tract)

Magnesium Tincture (calming and replenishing)

High Quality CBD Oil (calming/balancing/anxiety)

COFFEE ALTERNATIVE: MUD/WTR™

This product is amazing. Nine supplements in one, great for energy and focus, with 1/8th the amount of caffeine as compared to coffee. This wonderful alternative allows me to still have that warm morning ritual without the jitters, and is the only replacement that I have found to give me the necessary energy to start my day. In addition, this company's mission is mental health based, so it is truly a win-win in my book.

MUD/WTR™ INGREDIENTS
Masala Chai (energy/blood pressure/bloating)
Cocoa (blood pressure/inflammation)
Lion's Mane (depression/anxiety)
Chaga (anti-aging)
Reishi (fatigue)
Cordyceps (energy)
Turmeric (inflammation)
Cinnamon (hormonal balancing)
Himalayan Salt (replenishing)

Added in:
Collagen Powder (less wrinkles never hurt/
immunity/energy)
Ashwagandha Powder (calming/mood)
Creamer of your Choosing (nondairy if possible)

GREEN JUICE COCKTAIL
Sorry, but these ingredients have to be organic... too many chemicals if not.
Celery
Lemon

Ginger

Cucumber

Green Apples

ALL OF THE WOO-WOO MAGIC

If you aren't into any of that woo-woo "pseudoscience" stuff, well, now is the time to start, my friend. If you believe in energy, and that we are all energy-based beings floating around this universe together, then you have to at least be open and curious about the idea that the earth and its people, minerals, rocks, plants, and cells all are connected to that energy. We are all in this together and acknowledging the possibility that our earth provides energy healing can be a very helpful resource in finding your joy. About the time I was undergoing holistic therapy and PSYCH-K balances, I kept getting a pull to research essential oils and crystals. I was seeing them around me at every turn and witnessing how magical they were in the sense of well-being and health. I knew that synthetic smells (candles) gave me a headache and that crystals were some of the prettiest things I had ever laid eyes on. And in my Projector Lindsay fashion, I researched them to no end. I found that the oils from the earth and from plants could heal, could lift a mood, and could ultimately bring me and my family more joy. Smelling an uplifting scent all day as opposed to a synthetic chemical can be life changing. Dabbing oil on my son's chest when he was worked up calmed him down. Using them in my cleaning products make me loathe the process less. Sleeping next to my diffuser significantly helped my rest and increased my well-being. I also found out that every crystal, big or small, polished or raw, was tied to a very meaningful and purposeful body and mind benefit. By adding them to my workspace, my son's bedroom, my travel bag, and overall life, I noticed a change in my health and happiness. Part science, part magic, and part placebo; a powerful tool, nonetheless. I invite you to experiment with the high-quality essential oils available to you and to play with all of the magical crystals. Have fun and enjoy the process.

WHO CARES what other people say or think! This is YOUR life, YOUR journey, and YOUR JOY.

Be selfish, become aware, acknowledge, play, and release.

You got this momma.

A Letter to my Heroes

Dear Mommas,

I see you; I feel you; and you are not alone, my friend. You are doing the absolute best you can, within your level of consciousness, with the situations, life and circumstances that you are being dealt. You are an amazing person, human being and mother and although you may not see or feel it, there is JOY bubbling beneath the surface, ready to explode. It's within all of us. I invite you to be open and curious and to take your time. Choose one section of this book that is really speaking to you and start there. Your journey is so very unique and must be honored. Begin experimenting with what lights you up and move slowly. Notice how each layer brings more light and love to the surface, and how you feel as you move through the experiment. Good and bad. Praise yourself along the way. Reward yourself with more self-care and more inner knowing. You are doing a great job. Give yourself some slack, love. Surround yourself with people that care and that are fully supportive of your journey. Rid yourself of those people and things that don't serve. Life is short and the time is now. Your power lies in this very moment and you are extremely capable of manifesting JOY.

You've got this. You are my hero.

With so much love and light,
(and maybe a little Xanax sprinkled in)
Lindsay

CPSIA information can be obtained
at www.ICGtesting.com
Printed in the USA
LVHW011227130421
684341LV00021B/1006